HIGH BLOOD PRESSURE

HIGH BLOOD PRESSURE

PETER J. LEWIS MD, MRCP(UK).

Consultant Physician to the Hypertension Clinic,
Hammersmith Hospital, London

CHURCHILL LIVINGSTONE
EDINBURGH LONDON MELBOURNE AND NEW YORK 1981

CHURCHILL LIVINGSTONE
Medical Division of the Longman Group Limited

Distributed in the United States of America by
Churchill Livingstone Inc., 19 West 44th Street, New York,
branches and representatives throughout
the world.

First published 1981

ISBN 0 443 02301 8

British Library Cataloguing in Publication Data
Lewis, Peter J
High blood pressure. - (Patient handbook
series).
1. Hypertension
I. Title   II. Series
616.1'32   RC685.H8   80-41097

Printed in Singapore by Ban Wah Press

PREFACE

In Britain today about 4 million people suffer from the effects of high blood pressure. Probably only half of that number are aware that anything is wrong and only half are receiving treatment. At the very lowest estimate about one person in twenty has a blood pressure which warrants treatment.

However, for many patients high blood pressure is a confusing condition. How can it not be a disease and yet not require treatment? How can I have high blood pressure and yet feel quite well? Why must I take tablets when I have no symptoms? This book aims to answer such questions not as a substitute for the advice patients may get from their own doctors but rather to provide background information about this important subject.

London, 1981   P J L

CONTENTS

CONTENTS

1. WHAT IS HIGH BLOOD PRESSURE?

High blood pressure is a medical condition in which the patient, although not ill, is at risk of developing heart disease, kidney failure and stroke. The diagnosis is made by finding persistently high blood pressure on several occasions.

Is it difficult to be certain that a patient has high blood pressure?

Yes. There is a tremendous difference between having *a* high blood pressure and having high blood pressure! Anyone, even a perfectly normal individual, will have a high blood pressure after having run for a bus or having had a row with a traffic warden. However, in those patients with the condition of high blood pressure, blood pressure is up consistently and persistently. The problem is that blood pressure is a very variable thing much influenced by activity and mental state. This makes the evaluation of a single high blood pressure measurement very difficult. In those patients who have suffered from high blood pressure for some time, the doctor may find other changes on physical examination such as a more forceful beat of the heart and narrowing of the small blood vessels at the back of the eye.

Why is high blood pressure important?

High blood pressure is important because it is an underlying cause of much heart disease and most strokes. These conditions are very common causes of death in Western countries today. High blood pressure is particularly important because patients with this condition usually have no symptoms and may be quite unaware that anything is wrong. Thus, although treatment is effective, many do not seek it and may even feel disinclined to accept it when it is offered. Doctors treating high blood pressure think people ought to be more aware of the problem. High blood pressure is public health enemy number one.

Is high blood pressure a disease?

High blood pressure is not a disease in the usual sense of the term. With, say chicken pox, one either has the disease or one has not. However, blood pressure is a quantity. Everyone has a blood pressure just as everyone has a weight or a height. The difference between those with high blood pressure and those with normal blood pressure is one of quantity, not of kind. We all know that people vary in height; most of us are of average height and a few individuals are either very tall or very short. The same consideration applies to blood pressure. Having high blood pressure or being tall cannot be regarded as diseases but they are conditions which predispose people to other conditions. Having high blood pressure is important because it predisposes to heart attack and stroke. Being very tall is much less of a problem — it only predisposes to banging one's head on doorways!

How is blood pressure measured?

Blood pressure is measured by blowing up a rubber cuff around the upper arm and observing how much pressure is needed in the cuff to stop blood flowing through the artery beneath. Flow in the artery is detected by listening to it through a stethoscope. Blood pressure measurements are recorded as two numbers, e.g. 120/80. The first number is called the systolic pressure and represents the peak of pressure in the artery which is produced when the heart beats. The second number is the lowest pressure in the artery which occurs between heart beats and is called the diastolic pressure. The units of blood pressure are millimetres of mercury (mmHg) as the height of a mercury column is usually used to measure the pressure in the arm cuff.

What is hypertension?

Hypertension is merely the technical term for the condition of high blood pressure.

How high is high blood pressure?

It is difficult to give a definite answer to this because blood pressure normally increases with age. The World Health Organisation has suggested that a blood pressure of 140/95 or more at rest is abnormal at any age but this is just a guideline and it is not interpreted too strictly.

Are there different sorts of high blood pressure?

Yes. There are many different ways of dividing up patients with the condition. The most obvious is to divide patients up into severe high blood pressure, those in whom the condition is moderate and those in whom it is mild. Some patients develop complications of the condition in which some damage occurs as a result of the blood pressure. Hence complicated or uncomplicated blood pressure. Most patients have 'essential' hypertension which means that no underlying cause for the condition has been found as opposed to others who have 'secondary' hypertension, meaning that their blood pressure is raised due to some underlying problem such as kidney disease. High blood pressure may also be benign or malignant. Malignant hypertension is explained on page 6. However, in practical terms, perhaps the most important classification of patients with high blood pressure is into treated and untreated. It is this which makes the most difference.

How common is high blood pressure?

High blood pressure is very common and there is no doubt that it is one of the major causes of chronic ill health and premature death in the British Isles today. Using the very strictest of definitions, at least 3 per cent of the British population over the age of 40 has persistent high blood pressure and would benefit from medical treatment. These individuals have moderate to severe hypertension and treating them would reduce the number of strokes and heart attacks in the community. But this is not the end of the problem. There is an even larger group of individuals with only mild hypertension, that is to say with a diastolic blood pressure of between 95 and 105 mmHg where it is likely that treatment would be beneficial. This might mean that as many as one in five middle-aged men and women would benefit from having their blood pressure treated.

It has been estimated that high blood pressure is directly responsible for 15,000 deaths each year in Britain and is an underlying cause of 250,000 deaths from strokes, heart disease and kidney disease. In numerical terms, hypertension is a more important health problem than smoking or road accidents. Fortunately it is also a treatable condition.

How long has high blood pressure been known about?

High blood pressure has a relatively short history. It was only in 1905 that a reliable method of measuring blood pressure was developed. Thereafter, many different studies have shown that those people with the highest blood pressures live less long than those with normal blood pressures and that deaths from heart attack, kidney disease and stroke are the main causes of death for people with hypertension. It was only 30 years ago, in 1951, that the first effective drugs were introduced for the treatment of high blood pressure and only in the last 10-15 years that really acceptable drugs have made the treatment of hypertension a relatively straightforward and simple matter.

Is high blood pressure different in men and women?

Women fare slightly better than men as far as blood pressure is concerned. Hypertension is more common in young men than in young women but the incidence increases as women get older. After the menopause hypertension is more common in women than in men. Men suffer more heart attacks than women but this trend is tending to alter with women catching up. The incidence of stroke and kidney failure is about the same in men and women. Having high blood pressure can be a real problem to young women as it debars them from using the contraceptive pill and makes pregnancy a more difficult affair. Treatment of high blood pressure is equally effective in men and women.

How is blood pressure influenced by age?

In most societies and racial groups, blood pressure increases as people get older so that the criteria for high blood pressure are different for different age groups. A blood pressure which would be abnormal in a teenager, may be quite normal in a man of 70. For this reason it is difficult to give hard and fast definitions of what is a high blood pressure and what is a normal blood pressure. A rule of thumb which has served well in the past is that the systolic blood pressure should be no more than '100 plus your age', e.g. for someone aged 40, not more than 140.

Do children have high blood pressure?

Secondary hypertension, that is blood pressure caused directly by another disease, particularly of the kidneys, certainly occurs in children and is treated by paediatricians with the same sort of drugs as are used in adults. Essential or constitutional high blood pressure can also be recognisable in childhood and adolescence. There is evidence that those primary school children whose blood pressure is higher than their class mates will continue to stay ahead of their fellows in this regard when they become adult. This consistency of blood pressure through life, individuals tending to remain in the middle, low or high range of pressure is called tracking.

What is malignant hypertension?

In the days before effective drugs for blood pressure, it was observed that some patients with hypertension developed an acute debilitating illness and died in a few months. Microscopic examination of the small blood vessels in the heart, kidney and brain of these patients showed evidence of necrosis or cell death. It appeared as if the small blood vessels of the body became suddenly unable to take the strain of the increased pressure and started to break up. This syndrome of very high blood pressure and death within a few months could be diagnosed by examining the back of the eye with an ophthalmoscope. At the back of the eye small blood vessels are easily visible as they run over the retina. When malignant hypertension occurs, break-up of these small blood vessels can be seen. Nowadays, cases of malignant hypertension still occur but the condition need no longer be fatal as the blood pressure can be lowered with drugs and after a period of time, healing of the small blood vessels takes place. In patients who have been treated adequately with drugs, the condition of malignant hypertension hardly ever occurs.

Do any particular groups suffer more from hypertension?

Yes, hypertension is particularly common and severe in black people. In the United States high blood pressure is 4 times more common in black Americans than in whites. The mortality from hypertension is 10 times higher in young blacks than in young whites. In Britain this racial difference in the severity of high blood pressure is not as marked but it has been frequently observed that West Indians do have a high incidence of severe hypertension and they suffer badly from the complications of the condition.

Not surprisingly, West Indians are more aware of high blood pressure as a problem and often more knowledgeable about it than white patients. It is not known what the basis of this racial difference is. Numerous theories have been put forward and as with any other racial difference it is difficult to discuss the problem without political overtones. It may be that the tendency of black people to develop hypertension is purely inherited. Others have argued that black people are often economically under-privileged and therefore lead more stressful lives. Whatever the reason for the problem, studies in our clinic at Hammersmith Hospital show that once on treatment for high blood pressure West Indians do just as well as white patients.

Are there doctors who specialize in high blood pressure?

Hypertension is such an important and common problem that in many centres special clinics have been established to help diagnose and treat the condition. The specialists responsible for these clinics are usually physicians or 'medical doctors'. These doctors often have other interests, usually in kidney or heart disease, or occasionally in clinical pharmacology. However, many patients with high blood pressure do not need hospital treatment and may prefer to be looked after by their own family doctors.

2. WHAT EFFECTS DOES HIGH BLOOD PRESSURE HAVE?

High blood pressure literally 'takes years off your life'. These years are lost due to premature death from a variety of causes. In addition, high blood pressure can precipitate a variety of illnesses of the heart, kidneys and circulation. However, up until the moment one of these effects supervenes, the patient may be totally unaware of anything being wrong. For this reason hypertension has been called the 'silent killer'.

How much does high blood pressure affect life expectancy?

Blood pressure is the best single predictor of life expectation which is known. The reduction of life expectation, even with modest elevations of blood pressure, is very considerable. These conclusions are largely based on a huge body of information gathered by life assurance companies in America. In the 20 years between 1935 and 1954 life assurance companies in the U.S.A. required a medical examination and a blood pressure reading from every prospective client. Being life insurance companies, they also know very precisely when their insured clients died and of what they died. Because of this they were in an ideal position to relate the blood pressures of their insured lives to their mortality. These statistics, based on the results of 4 million life policies, provide a very clear message: the higher the blood pressure, the shorter the life.

It is possible to use these statistics so that an individual patient may apply them to his own case. We may take, for example, the life expectation of a young man of 35. If this man has a blood pressure of 120/80 or less, then he can expect, statistically, to live to the age of 76. If, however, the man's blood pressure is slightly elevated at 140/95, he can expect to die 8 years earlier at the age of 68. If the initial blood pressure was still higher, but still not greatly elevated at 140/100, his life expectancy would be only 60 years, a net loss of 16 years of life. These are really huge differences in life expectancy for very modest elevations of blood pressure, still in the mild range when even today we would hesitate to treat the patient. In human terms they are the difference between enjoying retirement or not, seeing one's grandchildren grow up or not, and doubling the length of widowhood.

Women fare slightly better in all this. They tend to have a longer life expectancy anyway and the effect of high blood pressure is correspondingly reduced. Nevertheless, the same message still applies. The higher the blood pressure, the shorter the life. The accompanying illustration shows some further figures for men and women aged 45 and 55 showing how life expectancy is directly related to the initial blood pressure. Incidentally, the blood pressures quoted here were ones taken at a single life insurance examination. It is likely that if the blood pressure had been taken on several occasions, a more representative blood pressure would have been obtained and the correlation would have been even better.

How are these reductions in life expectancy brought about?

The causes of death in patients with high blood pressure are most commonly heart attack, stroke and kidney failure. Stroke is six times more common in patients with moderately elevated blood pressure and heart attack is about three times more common. Overall, however, there are more deaths from heart attack than from stroke. Patients with very high blood

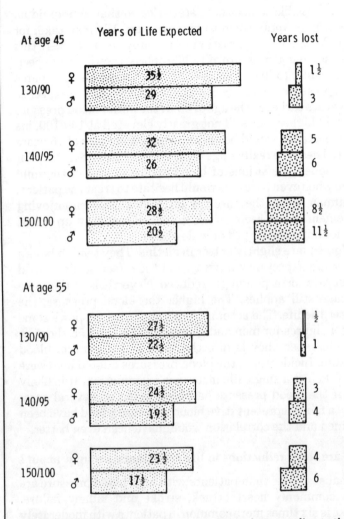

Life expectation for men and women aged 45 and 55 according to their blood pressure at that age. The higher the blood pressure the lower the expectation of life and the greater the years of expectation lost. Men have lower life expectancy than women at all ages and pressures.

10

pressure tend to die from malignant hypertension or from progressive kidney failure.

What symptoms does high blood pressure cause?

Many patients who are told they have hypertension are confused because they feel perfectly well and are convinced there must be some mistake. In popular mythology having high blood pressure is associated with a lot of precise symptoms, namely headache, dizziness, tenseness and anxiety. Some patients describe how they can 'feel the pressure going up' by sensations in their head. The fact is that high blood pressure, unless very severe and causing secondary problems, does not cause any symptoms. High blood pressure must be a very uncommon cause of headache. When headache is really due to raised blood pressure it is worse on lying down and particularly severe in the morning on waking.

What symptoms bring hypertension patients to their doctors?

Usually high blood pressure is found as an incidental finding when patients consult their doctors for an unrelated problem. After 3 years in our hypertension clinic when his blood pressure was under excellent control, one man complained to me that he still had his bunion which is what he had consulted his doctor about in the first place! Unfortunately not all patients do have cause to visit their doctors with bunions or it is possible that some may do so and not get a routine blood pressure check. These individuals may have their high blood pressure for years without knowing it and eventually present with a complication which could have been avoided if early diagnosis and treatment had been undertaken. Opticians also perform a very useful service in detecting high blood pressure which can show up as changes in the blood vessels at the back of the eye.

What complication can bring a patient to the doctor?

High blood pressure is often first found when a patient has a heart attack or a stroke or an attack of heart failure which presents usually as intractable shortness of breath, particularly at night. Other presentations occur with angina, that is to say pain in the chest on exertion caused by narrowing of the coronary arteries which supply oxygen to the heart. This late presentation is a tragedy because prevention is always more effective than trying to cure patients after they have developed these complications.

What about nose bleeds?

Traditionally nose bleeds, especially in people over 50, are associated with high blood pressure. These nose bleeds are often copious and the patient may become really alarmed which leads to an even higher blood pressure and more severe blood loss. For some reason patients with nose bleeds often lie down, snuffling and choking. What they should really do is sit up and pinch the nose firmly between finger and thumb, breathing through the mouth and holding a basin in the lap to catch the blood. If this manoeuvre does not work after 10-15 minutes, then the nose needs to be packed and this needs a visit to the hospital casualty department. It is one to two weeks after recovery from the nose bleed that the blood pressure needs to be checked.

Can one have high blood pressure and not know it?

Certainly. This is usually the situation. It is because of this difficulty that various attempts have been made to screen the population for high blood pressure. Various schemes have been tried. One of the most successful schemes was a 'supermarket screen' carried out in the U.S.A. and copied elsewhere. Realising that the supermarket was the place most often visited by the active middle-aged population who had most to benefit from high blood pressure treatment, hypertension doctors set up a booth in a supermarket and invited people in for a free blood pressure examination. Recently machines which automatically measure blood pressure have been appearing in stations and shops. In this way, people can check their blood pressures as easily as they can check their weight. Regrettably, the British Medical Association has condemned these machines on the grounds that they are meddlesome and might alarm patients. In my opinion, anything which takes a patient to his doctor to have his blood pressure checked cannot be a bad thing and I am all in favour of these machines. I am also in favour of patients taking their own blood pressure which is quite a simple thing to do. Machines for measuring blood pressure can be bought by mail order.

Can one have high blood pressure and never come to any harm from it?

This certainly can happen. Some patients seem to have a great resistance to high blood pressure and despite running high blood pressures for years they never have a stroke nor develop any other complications. Unfortunately these patients are rather rare and it is impossible to pick them out from the generality of patients where the higher the pressure the more the complications. All risks are really a statistical gamble after all. Almost everyone claims to have known or have heard about someone who smoked like a chimney, drank like a fish and lived to be a hundred. Unfortunately for every one of these fortunate individuals there must be many more who paid the price. So it is with blood pressure.

Is low blood pressure ever a problem?

Usually we regard low blood pressure as a blessing. Certainly the statistics show that the lower the blood pressure the longer the life. One of my colleagues' blood pressures is so low, 80/40, that I suspect he will live to be a 100. Occasionally low blood pressure can cause faintness and collapse but only if the pressure has dropped rapidly as occurs sometimes after an overdose of blood pressure tablets or after bleeding.

Some medical conditions like Parkinson's disease or Addison's disease are associated with a low blood pressure but there are other obvious features to these conditions. If one has low blood pressure and no other problems one can be very thankful.

Is high blood pressure life threatening?

A patient with hypertension is certainly at risk of dying from the condition. If adequately treated this risk is minimised. However, patients with high blood pressure can die of the condition without ever realising they had it. Such tragic presentations occur, for example, when a patient with undetected hypertension has a massive stroke and dies. I remember well the case of an apparently fit middle-aged man who was refereeing a country rugby match. During the second half he spotted a foul and blew his whistle. He ran over to the offender and began organising a penalty kick. Suddenly he stopped in mid-sentence and collapsed to the ground. He died a couple of hours later having never regained consciousness. At a postmortem examination it was found that he had had severe hypertension for some time and had suffered a huge stroke. Here was a fit man with no symptoms, who had unfortunately never had the opportunity of having his blood pressure taken. Obviously during the excitement and physical exertion of the game, his blood pressure had soared still further and burst a blood vessel in his brain.

3. WHAT CAUSES HIGH BLOOD PRESSURE?

The cause of high blood pressure has been actively sought by medical researchers for the last 50 years and yet it would be fair to say that we really do not know what it is. A lot has been discovered about the way the blood pressure is regulated by the body and certain separate diseases have been identified which cause high blood pressure in man. However, these only affect about 3 per cent of all the patients with high blood pressure and the underlying reason why the majority of people with hypertension suffer from the condition is not known. It seems fairly certain that there is not a single underlying cause of hypertension such as a virus or lack of a specific enzyme. Most doctors now believe that human hypertension is mainly due to genetic factors and that blood pressure is an inherited characteristic rather like height. Of course this still begs the question of which mechanisms of blood pressure control are being over-activated by the inheritance mechanism.

Have animal experiments shown any likely cause for the condition?

The most interesting information to come out of animal experiments on high blood pressure is, to my mind, that animals can be bred selectively to have either high or low blood pressure. Furthermore animals can be bred to be either resistant or susceptible to having strokes when they have

15

high blood pressure. This focuses on genetics and makes it less likely that we will find a single cause of high blood pressure in man. It is particularly interesting that laboratories in different parts of the world, for example in New Zealand, in Tokyo, in New York and in Milan have each produced rats with high blood pressure by selective breeding. However, the high blood pressure in each of these different strains of rats depends on different mechanisms. In one strain it is salt handling which is deficient, in another the kidney is responsible and in yet another the nervous system is overactive. This supports the belief that hypertension is a condition with many different causes and each patient may have a different collection of problems. In one patient stress may predominate, in another salt intake, in another a kidney problem and in another some as yet undefined cause.

Does high blood pressure run in families?

Very much so. The tendency to develop hypertension is very strongly influenced by inheritance. Most patients with the commonest essential form of high blood pressure have at least one parent whose blood pressure is elevated.

Will my children have high blood pressure too?

Children of patients with high blood pressure do have an increased risk for developing the condition but this is only a statistical risk and many of them will have quite normal blood pressure. The tendency for the blood pressure of children to be similar to those of their parents might of course be due to some characteristic of the home they share and the diet they eat rather than due to inheritance. However, studies on the blood pressure of adopted children show that there is no such tendency for the blood pressure to resemble that of the adoptive parent, so it seems clear that this influence is indeed due to inheritance. Interestingly, the blood pressures of husbands and wives are more often similar than would be expected by chance. It has been suggested that this is because blood pressure has some correlation with personality and this similarity of blood pressure comes about because people of similar temperament are attracted to one another.

Can high blood pressure be the sign of underlying disease?

Most patients with high blood pressure have no cause for their raised pressure, even when they are very carefully investigated. However, a few individuals do have some underlying problem. Most commonly this is some form of kidney disease which can consist of a persistent urinary infection, stones in the kidney, nephritis, or occasionally narrowing of an artery to the kidney. There are other rare causes of high blood pressure such as congenital narrowing of the aorta or benign tumours of the adrenal gland which secrete an excess of blood pressure-raising hormones. All these problems are relatively uncommon and show up with quite simple investigations such as the urine and blood tests commonly done when high blood pressure treatment is first started. High blood pressure is not associated with any more sinister illnesses such as cancer or leukaemia. Indeed the mortality from such diseases seems to be slightly lower in patients with hypertension, possibly because patients with high blood pressure are under closer medical supervision than the population as a whole.

How does kidney disease cause high blood pressure?

The kidney is a very important organ in the regulation of blood pressure. It controls the amount of salt and water in the body and in some types of high blood pressure it is this function which is important. More commonly, however, it is the secretion of a hormone called renin by the kidney which causes a rise in blood pressure. Renin was first discovered in 1898 but we are still having arguments about its role in blood pressure control. Certainly in some patients with narrowed arteries to one kidney it is the secretion of renin by the compromised kidney which pushes up the blood pressure, at least initially. There are now several drugs can directly counteract the effect of renin.

Can my blood pressure be due to stress?

There is no doubt that stress can raise a person's blood pressure. Blood pressure varies greatly with different activities and is lowest when a person is resting quietly unworried, unstressed and quiet. Even asking a person to perform mental arithmetic causes quite a dramatic rise in blood pressure. Painful stimuli, anxiety, or apprehension (all unfortunately quite common experiences in a medical consulting room) can also raise blood pressure. This short term effect of stress is undisputable. However, it is a big step from this to suggest that the condition of hypertension, by which we mean a sustained consistent elevation of blood pressure, is caused by prolonged stress. It may be but it is difficult to prove. Several investigators have shown that prolonged social stress seems to be associated with elevations of blood pressure. For example, when primitive rural people emigrate to industrial cities leaving their traditional way of life and joining the bottom rung of a competitive urban community, then their blood pressure consistently rises. When a whole community is westernised such as happened in the South Sea Islands, their pattern of blood pressure also becomes Westernised in that the blood pressure rises and they show the Western pattern of increasing blood pressure with increasing age. However, by themselves these studies do not prove the case because many other factors are involved in Westernisation and urbanisation. Diet is one such obvious factor and one obvious effect of westernisation is obesity.

Being overweight also predisposes to high blood pressure and city dwellers do tend to become fat.

Stress means different things to different people. Some individuals thrive on activity and competition while others become progressively more strained. When individuals are first diagnosed as having high blood pressure they tend to look for causes and reasons. They often complain that the last year has been a particularly stressful one for them with a change of job, a car accident, their daughter's examinations, etc. Some of these impressions may be quite misleading as present stress is always more real and pressing than other events in the past, now thankfully forgotten. Of course, what the patient is trying to say is that he believes his blood pressure would be quite normal if he led a stress-free existence. Maybe it would but this is impossible to prove and in any case a stress-free existence is an unattainable ideal. It would also be pretty boring. What we have to do in treating high blood pressure is to enable a patient to cope with his normal existence, stress and all.

Is there a hypertensive personality?

Many people have the image of somebody with high blood pressure as agressive, ambitious, competitive and impatient. Some years ago, American researchers coined the phase 'Type A personality'. People with a type A personality have a strong sense of 'time urgency'. They are forceful, rapid and emphatic. They do everything faster than most people and their entire existence, whether work or pleasure, is a race against time. The researchers claimed that 70 per cent of patients suffering a heart attack have a type A personality. Ranged against the type A is the type B personality, with the inverse of these characteristics. Type Bs have no time urgency, they are patient and they enjoy their leisure. The more engaging type B person likes winning but plays for fun. Type Bs have fewer heart attacks and live longer.

Unfortunately these two stereotypes seem to be fictional

characterisations. Occasionally one meets an individual who fits the stereotype but more often human beings are a mixture of these different characteristics. Patients with high blood pressure are no exception to this. In my experience, high blood pressure strikes the meek and mild with about the same frequency as it does the bold and assertive.

Is high blood pressure related to diet?

Diet is important in high blood pressure in two main ways. There is undoubtedly a strong correlation between over-weight and high blood pressure. Patients who are obese are more often hypertensive and when they diet and lose weight they have a corresponding reduction in their blood pressure. In some cases, this reduction in blood pressure can be really dramatic and can make the difference between the need for drug treatment or not. Losing weight is terribly difficult. Patients with obesity often complain at great length that they really eat very little indeed. Unfortunately, it does seem to be true that some overweight individuals are very efficient at converting the calories they eat into fat. Nevertheless there is no wonder cure for this situation and in order to lose weight patients must eat less. There is no reason why patients with high blood pressure should not do this by going on some 'fad' diet, be it all steak, all bananas, or all yogurt. For successful weight loss one often needs the novelty element which these diets provide.

The other aspect of diet which is important in high blood pressure is more difficult. It is the question of whether high blood pressure is influenced by the amount of salt in the diet. Here we enter upon an area of tremendous controversy. On the one hand we have authorities who believe that salt intake is totally irrelevant to blood pressure and on the other we have researchers who believe that an excessive salt intake is the main reason why patients develop high blood pressure. Certainly, there are strains of rats whose blood pressure is very sensitive to the amount of salt they eat, even within the normal dietary range. The amount of salt we eat in our diet is tending to increase. Modern convenience foods tend to mask their low quality with a high salt content to give them a satisfying taste. Crisps and nuts push up our salt intake and those of our children. The evidence that this increase in salt intake has any deleterious effect is rather tenuous. What we do know is that if salt intake is reduced very greatly then blood pressure will fall. Before drug treatment became available in the 1950s, salt restriction was the only effective way of reducing blood pressure and some patients owed their lives to this manoeuvre. Unfortunately, however, the salt content of an effective low salt diet must be very low. A very low salt content makes food impalatable.

What is not known is whether reducing the salt content of the diet by about half (coming down incidentally to the salt intake eaten by our ancestors) has any beneficial effect. Some authorities think it does. Certainly it seems a little illogical to allow patients with high blood pressure to eat whatever quantities of salt they like and then treat them with salt eliminating drugs. As so often with these things, a compromise seems indicated. We usually advise patients with high blood pressure to modify their diet slightly by not adding salt to food when it is being cooked, to avoid highly salted products and not to add any salt to their meals.

Finally there is one extremely uncommon cause of high blood pressure which doctors and patients often forget about. Over-consumption of liquorice can cause high blood pressure. In order to produce this effect one has to eat a great deal of liquorice but there are many cases recorded of patients who do just this. Apparently eating liquorice can be a sort of compulsive addiction. Some people eat over a pound of liquorice every day. Do you?

Does anyone ever grow out of high blood pressure?

Patients commonly hope that after a course of treatment

their blood pressure will become normal and nothing further need be done. It is very hard for someone to accept the fact that they have a condition which will probably require treatment for a very prolonged period and probably indefinitely. Most medical conditions are after all limited by time and do not persist indefinitely. Unfortunately, this does not seem to be the case with high blood pressure. What sometimes does happen, however, is that after some months or even years on drugs for high blood pressure, the patient becomes more sensitive to the drugs and the dose or even the number of different treatments can be reduced. Some patients who have taken small doses of drugs for years and whose blood pressures have been very well controlled have had their drugs withdrawn. Unfortunately, over a period of months it was noted that their blood pressure crept inexorably upward to what it was before they were treated. The truth of the matter seems to be that if after a course of treatment the blood pressure remains normal on no treatment then probably the diagnosis was wrong in the first place. In other words the patient did not have true hypertension or sustained elevation of blood pressure.

4. WHAT ABOUT SPECIAL TESTS?

The reason for carrying out any special test is always to answer questions about a patients condition which careful physical examination does not reveal. In the case of patients with high blood pressure, special tests are arranged to answer two main questions.
1. Has the high blood pressure caused any damage to the patient's heart or kidney?
2. Is there any underlying cause for the patient's high blood pressure?

How do the tests reveal the state of the heart?

With prolonged untreated high blood pressure, the heart comes under increasing strain and as with any muscle which is exercised it tends to grow thicker. Hence in high blood pressure, the heart tends to enlarge. This enlargement can often be detected on physical examination but it can be more accurately assessed on an X-ray of the chest. Another routine test is the electrocardiogram, or e.c.g., which is simply a recording of the electrical activity of the heart. The recording is made from cuffs attached to the wrists and ankles. In patients who have had untreated high blood pressure for some time, the e.c.g. may show evidence of strain. In severe cases one may see evidence of previous small heart attacks which may have occurred unnoticed by the patient.

How is kidney function investigated?

We can tell how well the kidneys are working simply by examining the urine and the blood. One of the main pre-occupations of doctors in past centuries was to examine the urine, usually holding it up to the light. Nowadays urine analysis is a bit more scientific. A test paper dipped in the urine can tell us the amount of protein in it. When protein leaks into the urine, this is an early sign of kidney damage. Chemical analysis of the blood gives us a very precise indication about kidney function. If the kidneys are not working well, then waste products build up in the blood.

How are tests used to detect underlying causes of high blood pressure?

Underlying causes for high blood pressure are rather uncommon. Some of these rare causes will show up on routine blood analysis, still others, such as forms of congenital heart disease will be seen on the chest X-ray. However, the majority of rare causes of high blood pressure are due to abnormalities in the kidneys. The kidneys can be X-rayed using a special X-ray called an i.v.p. which stands for intra-venous pyelogram. In this test, an iodine-based dye is injected into a vein and this dye is avidly removed from the blood by the kidneys. As the dye is opaque to X-rays, the position and size of the kidneys show up well. Most abnormalities of the kidneys show up on an i.v.p. but in some cases more elaborate X-rays of the kidneys are indicated.

One other extremely rare cause of high blood pressure is a so-called phaeochromocytoma. This is a benign tumour of the adrenal gland which secretes adrenaline, a blood pressure raising hormone. Occasionally patients with small tumours of this sort present simply with high blood pressure. In order to detect these tumours which literally occur in fewer than 1 in a 1000 patients with high blood pressure, a screening test is often carried out in which the patient collects all the urine that he passes for 24 hours into a special bottle. Subsequently the amount of adrenaline in the urine is measured and in this way an adrenaline-secreting tumour can be detected.

Are all these tests really necessary?

It is quite true to say that if none of these tests were carried out the treatment for most patients would be very little altered. In some sense a lot of unnecessary tests are done because we know that the majority of them will prove normal. Some doctors specialising in hypertension do very few of these tests, reserving, for example, the i.v.p. for patients whose blood pressure is subsequently difficult to control. Others feel that every patient should have the benefit of an investigation which might reveal a treatable cause. In general the more that is known about a patient's condition, the better.

Do these tests need to be repeated?

Tests to determine the underlying cause of the blood pressure need only be done once. However, investigations on heart and kidney function are usually repeated at intervals. They supply a check on the patient's progress. For example, if the patient's heart enlarges despite treatment or his kidney function deteriorates, these are important signs that the treatment is not being properly regulated and changes will have to be made. Persistent normality or the reduction in heart size which often occurs is an encouraging sign. Most clinics ask patients to provide a sample of urine whenever they attend for check up. This is a most important simple screening test which can pick up kidney problems before they have progressed too far.

Will I need to go into hospital?

A few years ago it was quite usual for all patients with newly diagnosed high blood pressure to be admitted to hospital for a few days for investigation, assessment and initiation of appropriate treatment. Such routine admissions are now less frequent. The tendency is for all tests and initiation of treatment to be carried out in the out-patient department. We have come to realise that a hospital admission is an expensive luxury and since most tests can be carried out in the out-patient department, it is not strictly necessary. In some ways I regret this change because the initial admission to hospital certainly impressed the patient and made him or her more likely to take his condition seriously. No one wishes a patient with high blood pressure to adopt a 'sick role'. Nevertheless, patients who are never admitted to hospital seem to take their treatment less seriously. Another aspect is that there is certainly less time for careful explanations about the nature of hypertension in a busy out-patient clinic.

5. HOW IS HIGH BLOOD PRESSURE TREATED?

Several sorts of treatment can lower blood pressure. Just admitting a patient to hospital and confining them to bed can have a dramatic effect on the blood pressure, presumably by removing the individual from the stresses and strains of the outside world, resting him and providing him with a regular, undemanding existence. In a more trendy way, transcendental meditation can have a similar sort of effect. Changing a patient's diet can also lower his blood pressure, especially if the total amount of salt and food eaten are reduced and the patient loses weight.

However, we live in a real world and few hypertensive patients have the time or inclination to leave their families and lie in bed meditating over a salt-free salad. For the majority of patients the effective treatment of high blood pressure means the administration of drugs. The occasional patient can get away with losing weight, cutting his salt intake and leading a less stressful existence. However, for the majority of patients with raised blood pressure, drug treatment is essential and of benefit.

Is treatment necessary?

Any medical treatment carries with it possible risks and potential benefits. The decision to use the treatment involves some calculation of these quantities. The benefits offered to patients with high blood pressure are considerable. The aim of treatment is to keep the patient well, to prevent or delay the onset of heart, kidney and stroke complications and to restore a full life expectancy to the patient. These benefits are obviously long-term and greatest in those patients with very severe high blood pressure and the poorest outlook. For the young man with mild hypertension, who has only a statistical chance of losing five years from the end of his life in 50 years time, the benefits of taking tablets today may well be difficult to appreciate. In difficult cases the decision must be left to the patient. His doctor will be able to explain how he sees this balance of risk and benefit for the individual patient.

How effective is treatment?

With modern drugs it is possible to lower blood pressure in practically all patients and to completely normalise it in the majority. All this can be achieved with disabling side effects. In this sense then the drugs certainly do work. However, what is more important is whether lowering the blood pressure with drugs will bring the patient's prospects for life and health back to what they would have been if his blood pressure was naturally at that level. Several large-scale investigations have looked at this using the established method of assessing drug treatment, with a prospective controlled trial. In such a trial one group of patients will receive the drug treatment, while another precisely similar group of patients will receive dummy pills or placebos. Trials of the effect of blood pressure lowering tablets in hypertension have been carried out both in the United States and in Britain and for patients with moderate and severe high blood pressure a clear benefit has been shown from the active treatment. Patients taking the blood pressure lowering drugs had a much lower rate of complications, particularly strokes, than the patients who did not receive active treatment. There is also no doubt that patients who develop malignant hypertension have their lives saved by antihypertensive drugs. There remains some argument as to whether patients with very mild hypertension benefit from treatment. Obviously these patients have a lesser risk anyway from the condition so it is more difficult to demonstrate benefit. However, one large-scale trial in Australia has recently indicated that treatment is beneficial. Another recent trial from America has also come to the same conclusion. In Britain we have a huge trial being conducted by the Medical Research Council. This is investigating whether patients with mild hypertension benefit from treatment or not. It is due to report its results in 1981 or 1982.

Can surgery help?

Surgery is of very limited help in the treatment of high blood pressure. In the days before effective drugs were available for the treatment of hypertension, operations were sometimes done which involved cutting certain nerves to blood vessels in the hope of relieving constrictor influences. These sympathectomy operations were successful in a few patients but often the benefit was short-lived. This operation is now only very rarely performed. Nowadays only patients with adrenal tumours and kidney disease are considered for operation. These are all very rare conditions and for the generality of patients with high blood pressure surgery has nothing to offer.

What can I do to help myself?

The first thing to realise that if you have hypertension it is unlikely to be due to anything you have done or have not done. A man is not responsible for his own blood pressure. Having said that, there are some factors you can tackle in order to positively improve your chances of not having a heart attack, not having a stroke and not developing kidney disease. These factors with suggestions on how to tackle them are as follows:

1. *Blood pressure*. First and foremost make sure that your high blood pressure is properly investigated and properly treated. More than half of the patients who are told that they have high blood pressure eventually stop their treatment. The reason is usually apathy rather than any positive dislike of the drugs. Compliance with treatment is most important. The intermediate step of pretending to be compliant and yet not taking the tablet is also fairly common and wastes both your time and the doctors' time. Reducing high blood pressure is the single most important thing one can do to improve one's chances of health.

2. *Smoking*. All the complications of hypertension are greater in those patients who continue to smoke. It is not known why this should be but it is a fact. Smoking is a very important risk factor for coronary heart disease. The two factors of high blood pressure and smoking seem to combine together to be particularly virulent. Smoking, of course, is harmful in lots of other ways including promoting bronchitis and carcinoma of the lung.

3. *Overweight*. Being overweight is also a risk factor for having a coronary thrombosis and it conspires again with the high blood pressure to increase the risk. We all known that losing weight is even more difficult than giving up smoking but it has to be done.

4. *Lack of exercise*. Exercise is important in heart disease. In the 1950s London epidemiologists compared the coronary heart disease rate of drivers and conductors on London buses. This was a beautiful experiment because drivers and conductors work the same hours in the same place, the only difference being that drivers sit down and conductors run up and down stairs all day. Coronary heart disease mortality was twice as high in the drivers than in the conductors. Numerous other studies have shown that activity protects against coronary heart disease.

4. *Stress*. Stress is the conflict between what we want to do

and what we have to do. On this definition, it obviously begins in the cradle. Stress is difficult to measure and difficult to investigate. It is therefore one of those rare occasions when the modern physician is allowed to give his impressions. In my opinion, many patients with high blood pressure are under stress, and they can benefit from having this reduced. Paradoxically the discovery of high blood pressure can reduce their level of stress simply because the condition and its treatment gives them some excuse to withdraw from the particular race in which they were engaged.

Do I need to go to a specialist clinic?

When high blood pressure is first discovered patients are often referred to a specialist clinic for evaluation. After the initial investigations, which are described in Chapter 4, treatment can be started. Very often this is a smooth, uncomplicated process, and the patient can be referred back to his own doctor. In patients who have severe high blood pressure or in whom there are complications, it is often better for the patient to continue to attend the hospital clinic. Some hypertension clinics offer a purely consultative service while others like to take full charge of their patients and follow them up indefinitely. Unfortunately there are so many patients with hypertension that this cannot always be done.

How frequently will I need a check up?

After the initial investigations when a patient is established on treatment he or she will need to be seen only 3 or 4 times a year. However clinics are very flexible and if there is any complication or if the blood pressure is difficult to control patients are seen oftener. In the initial stages patients may need to come to the clinic every week.

What is the usual routine at a hypertension clinic?

It is obviously essential to record the blood pressure and this is done either by the doctor seeing the patients or by a nurse technician. Great care is taken to ensure that the patient is relaxed when the pressure is taken and it is normal to take the blood pressure when the patient is lying down and when they are standing up. This is because the drugs which are used to treat hypertension will have different effects in the two positions. Patients who attend the hypertension clinic are usually asked to provide a urine specimen as a quick check on kidney function. Most of the consultation at the hypertension clinic is concerned with adjusting the drug treatment to get optimum blood pressure control. For this reason patients must bring their tablets with them or some up to date record of their present medication. It is surprising how many patients neglect to take this obvious step. It is also common for patients to arrive at the hypertension clinic dressed in some elegant creation from which it takes at least 5 minutes to extract a bare arm for a blood pressure measurement.

6. WHAT ABOUT DRUGS?

Drugs for high blood pressure really only date from the 1950s when the first ganglionic blocking drugs were introduced. These drugs interfered with the nervous control of blood vessel constriction and were the first successful treatment for malignant hypertension. These drugs, which were such a breakthrough in their time, have now been superceded by a new generation of drugs. Today the physician has many effective treatments but the main ones fit into 5 categories: the diuretics, the beta blockers, the vasodilators, the central drugs and the adrenergic drugs. There are many different drugs in each category and a glossary of all the different drugs is included in the back of this book. Many patients find drug names very difficult. The situation is rather confusing because the names sound like gibberish and the doctor often calls each drug by its several different names. The names sound peculiar because they are based on the chemical structure of the drug. Each drug also has a trade name or sometimes two. Further complications arise because some tablets contain a combination of drugs. It is absolutely essential that the patient carries some written record of the drugs he is taking. Most clinics provide cards with this information on it and they should be brought up to date whenever any alteration is made. Do not be afraid to insist that this is done.

What are water tablets?

Water tablets are the common name for diuretic drugs. These

drugs have the effect, at least initially, of promoting urine formation. However, they are used to treat high blood pressure for another action, their power to relax the blood vessels in the body. Diuretics are one of the two 'mainstay' treatments for high blood pressure and almost all patients with hypertension will be given them at some time. Diuretics have been around for a long time (the first one having been introduced in about 1958) and they are very useful drugs. They work well, they hardly ever produce any symptoms for the patients to complain of, with the possible exception of increasing the frequency with which they have to pass urine. For this reason diuretics are almost always taken in the morning. If taken at night diuretics may force the patient to get up more frequently to pass urine.

Although diuretics rarely produce troublesome symptoms, over prolonged periods of time they can cause gout or diabetes so periodic urine and blood tests are carried out on patients taking these drugs. Another minor problem with diuretics is that they cause an increased loss of potassium in the urine. Usually this loss of potassium is not great and on a normal diet, which includes fruit, enough potassium is taken in to compensate. Sometimes, however, potassium supplements are given with the diuretics. These potassium supplements are usually in the form of Slow K tablets or fizzy potassium tablets. Unfortunately in order to provide enough potassium several of these pills are often needed. Some patients have to take 9 of them a day. Patients can often forget that fresh fruit and orange juice is a more pleasant way of taking potassium and is just as effective.

What are beta blockers?

Beta blockers are a modern British invention which have revolutionised hypertension treatment. They were invented during the 1960s at ICI and the first beta blocker, pro-pranolol or Inderal, has been around for about 15 years. These drugs, together with diuretics, are now the mainstay of hypertension treatment. There are about 8 or 10 of these drugs having a similar action and they are all known collectively as the beta blockers. They have this name because they block the action of adrenaline at the beta receptor, the receptor on the heart which increases heart rate during exertion or anxiety. Patients taking these drugs tend to have a slow heart rate. The drugs are very good at lowering blood pressure and most patients find them easy to accept. The side effects which sometimes occur are minor and include a tendency to develop cold hands and feet, particularly in the winter and particularly in ladies. Some patients complain of tiredness of their legs on prolonged exercise. However, in general it is difficult for a patient to tell whether they are on a beta blocker or on a dummy tablet, the ideal situation for a drug lowering blood pressure. Patients with asthma or severe bronchitis cannot tolerate beta blockers as they tend to make asthma worse.

What about other drugs?

The **central drugs**, reserpine, methyldopa and clonidine lower blood pressure by an action within the brain. These drugs have all been around for 10 to 20 years and were once the mainline drugs used for treating high blood pressure. Recently they have been displaced by the beta blockers because central drugs tend to produce slight tiredness or lethargy, presumably by an action on the brain similar to sedatives. However, this tiredness often wears off within a few weeks and many patients tolerate the drugs quite happily.

The **adrenergic drugs**, guanethidine, debrisoquine and bethanidine are another group of drugs which were invented 20-25 years ago. They too have been displaced by the beta blockers but some patients have taken them contentedly for many years. The main problems with these drugs are that the blood pressure is lower when the patient is standing up or exercising than when he lies down. Because of this, the patients may get dizzy on standing or alternatively are too hypertensive when they are lying down. It is these drugs also that have particularly interfered with male sexual function and given blood pressure tablets a bad name.

The vasodilators, prazosin, hydralazine, minoxidil, are drugs which have an action directly on blood vessels. This group of drugs is now enjoying a resergence of popularity and patients often take a combination of one of these drugs plus a beta blocker plus a diuretic. The vasodilators have few side effects at the small doses in which they are now used but large doses sometimes cause a bulging headache immediately after the drugs are taken. Such a headache means that the dose should be reduced or spread out evenly over the day.

Why are several drugs often used together?

Using several drugs together is quite a deliberate policy on the doctor's part. In this way the side effects of each drug can be kept to a minimum by reducing the dose. The total dose of drug can also be reduced because each drug attacks the regulation of blood pressure at a different mechanism and the combined effect and a combined attack is more effective. The most usual combination is a diuretic with a beta blocker and a vasodilator. Many patients with mild hypertension, of course, only need one drug and nowadays the choice would usually be a diuretic or a beta blocker. Patients with very severe hypertension may end up on a long list of drugs as their blood pressure is very difficult to control. In this case it is particularly important that they should keep a clear understanding of their treatment if they are not to take the tablets incorrectly.

What side effects can be expected from these drugs?

The side effects commonly encountered for each of the different types of drugs have already been described (p. 00). Perhaps the most unusual side effect of taking treatment for high blood pressure and one that does not appear in any of the textbooks is the feeling of disquiet and resentment that any treatment may be necessary. Many patients starting treatment for uncomplicated hypertension simply cannot accept the fact that they need drugs. In our society drugs have a bad name. They stand for indulgence and weakness. 'I never so much as take an aspirin, doctor' is a common refrain which in reality means that 'I have been good and now you want me to be bad'. This unfortunate association of drug taking and weakness is difficult to overcome and patients are often very resentful about having to take drugs on a long-term basis. In these cases side effects due to the drug are particularly resented. The incidence of these side effects is fortunately really rather low, particularly for the beta blockers and diuretics but obviously side effects do occur from time to time.

However, hypertension doctors sometimes find it difficult to accept certain complaints as genuine side effects. We know that placebo or dummy tablets provoke a variety of side effects, even in perfectly rational individuals. These side effect sensations are not due to the tablet, which is inert but are due to the patient anticipating side effects and then seizing on any odd sensation which occurs and attributing it to the pill. Following this the patient unconsciously magnifies the sensation and begins to experience it each time he takes the pill. These pseudo side effects can be as real to the patient as a genuine effect but if a dummy pill is substituted for the active tablet, then the same side effect is seen, obviously imagined by the patient. These side effects are of this imagined sort. Particularly commonly patients imagine unsteadiness, bursting sensations in the head, tremulousness, nausea and sweating. Another feature of these pseudo side effects is their timing. Often the symptom is felt almost the instant the pill is taken, long before the drug can be absorbed and any real effect could be apparent.

37

What about alcohol and these drugs?

Alcohol and high blood pressure are not very importantly related. Alcohol withdrawal from an alcoholic sometimes precipitates a rise in blood pressure as the withdrawal symptoms come on. However, alcohol itself does not interfere with the action of any of the antihypertensive drugs and patients taking them need have no particular reason to change their drinking habits. Smoking is a much more important risk factor for people with high blood pressure than is moderate alcohol intake.

What about other drugs?

Certain other drugs do indeed interfere with blood pressure tablets and patients should consult their doctors before taking any other medication no matter how trivial. One such important interaction occurs with cold cures, capsules, powders and fruit flavoured potions which can be bought over the counter of the chemist. These remedies such as 'Medinight', 'Night nurse', 'Mucron tablets', 'Contac' capsules, etc, usually contain a drug based on adrenaline which is helpful in clearing up a blocked nose. These cold cures are really very effective. However in patients on adrenergic drugs they can cause a marked rise in blood pressure which can be dangerous. Drugs such as aspirin and paracetamol do not interfere with the action of antihypertensives and are safe for the hypertensive patient to take.

7. HOW WILL HYPERTENSION AFFECT MY LIFE?

Many people who are told they have high blood pressure find it extremely difficult to accept that there is really anything wrong. Now that high blood pressure is more commonly detected at an early stage, it is likely that the patient has no symptoms at all and feels perfectly well. A common reaction to being told that treatment is necessary is for the patient to angrily reject this. It is often easier for a patient to accept treatment if it is explained to him that hypertension is not a disease and that the treatment proposed is purely prophylactic and aimed at preventing trouble. Thus some of the initial problem is a psychological one rather than a physical one. Some patients reject the diagnosis, reject the treatment and defy nature to do its worst. Others adopt the sick role and start cultivating symptoms of headache and dizziness which they think appropriate to someone with high blood pressure. Fortunately, however, the majority of patients soon come to terms with the problem and accept treatment in a philosophical way, grateful that there is indeed some normalizing treatment for them. The psychological problems are often greater than those symptoms which arise from drug treatment, which at least so far as the diuretics and beta blockers are concerned, are almost undetectable. Patients with high blood pressure should be able to lead an almost normal life.

What about my job?

I cannot think of a single occupation which cannot be

successfully followed by a patient with uncomplicated hypertension who is taking appropriate treatment. Having said that, patients with severe or complicated hypertension are obviously at risk from developing such a sudden event as a heart attack. They would obviously, therefore, not be suitable for flying aircraft. The Aviation Authority would probably prevent them from doing so. However in more mundane occupations there are very few situations where people with high blood pressure cannot perform normally. It is unfortunately quite common for patients with high blood pressure who drive vehicles to be transferred to other work. This is probably unnecessary but if a supervisory job can be found for such people, then well and good. Heavy physical work is more difficult for men on beta blockers and patients on central drugs sometimes find difficulty with their work if this involves concentrated calculation or thought. However, for the majority of individuals having high blood pressure and taking treatment should not affect their work nor their prospects.

Can I get life insurance if I have high blood pressure?

Many life insurance companies weight the premiums on people with high blood pressure. As we have seen, they have good statistical evidence for doing this, as the higher the blood pressure, the less long the life expectancy. Nevertheless this was the case with high blood pressure before treatment became available and many life offices are taking a more realistic view and offering policies with very little weighting if the patient is taking effective antihypertensive treatment, is making good progress and is attending regularly for follow-up. Of course, a patient who is taking antihypertensive drugs will have a normal blood pressure when he is examined medically and if he does not declare that he is taking the drugs or that he has high blood pressure to the insurance doctor, then it may not be detected. A policy may then be issued without any loading. Of course such a manoeuvre on the patient's part amounts to fraud and a fraud which is very likely to come to light subsequently. This will invalidate the insurance policy and it would seem a more prudent and a more honest plan to make an open declaration to the insurance company and to shop around for a company that does not weight life insurances for uncomplicated treated hypertension.

What about sport?

The general advice here is to do what you can manage but not to overdo it. We certainly do not want to discourage patients with high blood pressure from taking exercise. However, during vigorous competitive sport such as sprinting, squash or rugby there may be tremendous surges of blood pressure and these are best avoided No hypertensive in his right mind would ever go in the boxing ring. However, other activities within reason are to be encouraged. The current jogging craze is probably fine for a hypertensive if it leads to him losing weight but again it is unwise for the hypertensive to push himself to the point of exhaustion.

Can I go abroad?

Certainly you may go abroad. However, you would be extremely wise to take a reasonable stock of your usual medication with you. You would be even wiser to pack these drugs in your hand baggage as airlines regularly lose suitcases. As a back-up take with you a note of the drugs you are currently taking. In hot climates the blood pressure falls lower than in cold climates so if you become dizzy, try reducing the dose of your tablets somewhat. If you are thinking of emigrating or going abroad for a long period of time, remember to look into the cost of medical care in your new country. If you have to buy the drugs, it may cost you several hundred pounds a year.

What about my sex life?

Having high blood pressure per se does not affect any part of the sexual performance. However, some of the older drugs used for treatment of hypertension, particularly the adrenergic neurone drugs, such as guanethidine, bethanidine and debrisoquine, did interfere with male sexual function. In men taking these drugs there was sometimes failure of ejaculation. The drugs themselves did not interfere with erection and so did not cause impotence. However, the drugs most commonly used today, diuretics and beta blockers are thought not to have any appreciable effect on sexual function. In this regard it might be mentioned, however, that patients on beta blockers occasionally complain of exceptionally vivid dreams. Sometimes the content of these dreams is rather explicitly sexual and a few patients find them upsetting.

Some patients worry about their blood pressure during intercourse, having read somewhere that sexual excitement can raise the blood pressure greatly. In fact the blood pressure rise during intercourse is not very great and is about equivalent to running up two flights of stairs so patients are unlikely to come to any harm on this account.

What if I run out of tablets?

Don't! If you do run out of tablets don't wait for a couple of weeks until your next visit to the clinic. Try and get some more as soon as possible from your GP, from the hospital outpatients, from the casualty department or from anywhere that will give you a prescription. It is a good plan to get your tablets regularly from the same pharmacy and then they may be able to help you out. Some types of drug are particularly dangerous when they are stopped suddenly. The most important of these is clonidine. If these tablets are stopped for 24 hours or more, it is quite common for the patient to feel most unwell with tremulousness and palpitation. Stopping beta blockers suddenly may also be hazardous.

Can I have an operation while on blood pressure tablets?

This is certainly possible. The usual drill is for the tablets to be continued right up to the operation and started again soon afterwards. It is particularly important to tell the anaesthetist and surgeon about your treatment, to bring your tablets with you to the hospital and to provide the house surgeon with a list of the drugs which you are on.

What about the dentist?

Show the dentist the list of the drugs that you are taking. It should make little difference to your treatment but the dentist may decide not to use local anaesthetic in which there is added adrenaline. Never agree to have a general anaesthetic in a dental surgery. If you need dental surgery under an anaesthetic this can be done at hospital.

8. WHAT ABOUT THE PILL AND PREGNANCY?

Having high blood pressure can debar a woman from taking the pill and make pregnancy much more difficult. Furthermore, both the pill and pregnancy can induce a rise in blood pressure.

Can the pill cause high blood pressure?

Yes. The pill can cause high blood pressure and this is why the blood pressure should be checked every 6 months or so in women who are taking it. If the blood pressure rises on the pill, it usually returns to normal when the pill is stopped but this is not always the case. It is thought that the pill unmasks a tendency for high blood pressure and in some cases the hypertension persists when the pill is withdrawn. Occasionally women who develop hypertension on the pill can be switched to the mini pill which consists of progesterone only but this is a less reliable means of contraception than the combined pill.

Can I take the pill if I have high blood pressure?

Opinions are divided about this. Usually women with high blood pressure are debarred from taking the pill as it has been found that the pill tends to increase still further the blood pressure in these women and this is very undesirable. Occasionally doctors prescribe the pill for such women and are prepared to increase the dose of antihypertensive drugs if necessary.

If I become pregnant will the tablets affect the baby?

There is no evidence that any of the tablets currently used for high blood pressure produce abnormalities in babies. Women who have high blood pressure sometimes have difficult pregnancies but it has been shown that drug treatment during the pregnancy actually helps the baby's chances of growth and survival. Women with high blood pressure are well advised to consult their doctors if they are thinking of starting a pregnancy so that the best combination of tablets can be arranged. Methyldopa is one drug which is frequently used during pregnancy and there is no evidence that it harms the baby. More recently, beta blockers have been given to pregnant women with good results. In early pregnancy the blood pressure falls considerably with a general relaxation of the blood vessels and so frequent changes in drug dosage are necessary for expectant mothers.

If I had high blood pressure when I was pregnant, will this trouble occur again?

There is a type of high blood pressure which only occurs in late pregnancy called pre-eclampsia. The origin of this condition is obscure but it is much more common in the first pregnancy than in subsequent pregnancies. The usual treatment is admission to hospital, bed rest, sedation and an early induction of the delivery. It seems that having pre-eclampsia does not predispose women to getting high blood pressure in later life when they are not pregnant and the chances are also that it will not recur in a second or subsequent pregnancy.

9. HOW DOES HYPERTENSION CAUSE HEART ATTACKS?

Heart attacks are due to blockage of one of the coronary arteries which are the blood vessels which supply the heart with oxygen. We do not know why the coronaries are particularly likely to these blockages but we do know a lot of things which predispose to such an event. These include high blood pressure, high cholesterol, smoking, being overweight and taking little exercise. High blood pressure damages blood vessels in some way and they become stiff and their lining becomes studded with pimply lumps called atheroma. These lumps often form the focus for thrombosis in which cells from the blood stick together. In patients with high blood pressure the heart is enlarged so the effects of any blockage of the coronary arteries are that much worse. On the other hand, there is more evidence that if a patient is taking a beta blocker at the time that he sustains a heart attack then the outcome is rather better than it would otherwise be.

What is a stroke and how does high blood pressure cause one?

A stroke, (abbreviated from 'stroke of God') is a sudden loss of power or sensation caused by haemorrhage or blood clot in the brain. The blood vessels most commonly affected in a typical stroke are in the centre of the brain where the motor or movement nerve fibres run and an upset here causes a weakness of arm and leg on one side, usually not both. Mercifully, strokes are usually painless as the brain itself has no inner sensation. The patient may become drowsy or even unconscious as a result of swelling after the injury. Usually some function returns gradually and most patients who have a stroke recover sufficiently well to be able to walk. A good rule is if there is any flicker of function in any apparently paralysed muscle 6 weeks after a stroke, then eventually some useful function will return to that muscle. Occasionally, however, the first stroke can prove fatal. Other disabling complications are loss or severe disturbance of speech. Often in these cases the patient knows what he wishes to say but cannot get the words out because the speech area of the brain is affected. Strokes on the right side affect speech in right handed people and strokes on the left side in left handed people can affect speech.

What actually happens in stroke is that a blow out occurs in a minute area of weakness in one of the central arteries of the brain. These little blow outs are called aneurysms and they can just be distinguished with the naked eye. The formation of these aneurysms is directly related to the height of the blood pressure and the length of time it has been elevated. Blow out of one of these aneurysms is also related to the blood pressure at the moment of the stroke. In both these ways treating blood pressure with drugs helps reduce the incidence of stroke.

A stroke can be a terribly disabling and degrading thing, reducing an independent and attractive person to a mute unhappy invalid who is a burden to his family. If it were solely the incidence of stroke which was reduced by treating blood pressure, then the treatment would be very worthwhile.

What is kidney failure?

The function of the kidneys is to remove impurities from the body which build up continuously as a result of normal body processes. Producing urine and secreting these impurities into it is an active process requiring a lot of energy. Functionally the two kidneys are a mass of closely packed blood vessels coiling around the tubules into which the urine is filtered. In high blood pressure, the blood supply to the kidneys is impaired and there is a progressive loss of kidney tubules. The kidneys actually shrink and gradually lose their capacity to excrete as much waste material as is produced by the body. At this point toxic materials start to build up in the blood and the patient is said to be in renal failure. The patient loses weight, becomes anaemic and acquires a characteristic lemon-yellow tinge to the skin. The patient feels unwell and may be nauseated. Unless checked, renal failure is a fatal condition, the only treatment being either a renal transplant or frequent dialysis on the kidney machine. Once any impairment of kidney function is detected treatment of raised blood pressure is absolutely vital if the disease is not to progress.

What is claudication?

Claudication is the technical term for the characteristic pain which patients suffer in the calves on walking if there is a blockage in the main arteries of the legs. The pain is due to not enough oxygen getting through to the calf muscles during exercise. It is indeed a form of cramp. Claudication is the result of arterial disease and again is largely due to the effects of high blood pressure but is also contributed to by smoking and the other risk factors which influence coronary heart disease.

10. THE FUTURE

It is always difficult to look ahead but the future is very much rosier for patients with high blood pressure now than it was 30 years ago. Then drugs for high blood pressure had only just been introduced and they had horrendous side effects. Patients on these early drugs could not stand upright without intolerably dizziness, had visual disturbances and they were terribly constipated. Because of these side effects, only the most dangerously ill patients could be treated. How different the situation is today. Now we have excellent drugs and because of this we are able to extend their benefits to more and more patients with mild hypertension. I suppose this trend will continue. The present tragedy is that treatment is just not getting through to a sufficient number of people. At present only about half of those with high blood pressure know that they have the condition and of those only about a quarter are being adequately treated. With better awareness of high blood pressure, I hope that these proportions will change and as a result we can look forward to a great reduction in strokes and heart attacks.

Are new drugs being developed?

Certainly. Research into antihypertensive drugs is one of the most active endeavours of the pharmaceutical industry. The development of beta blockers was a major breakthrough. Still new classes of drugs are likely to emerge. Ease of treatment is likely to improve in succeeding years and the ideal of a single tablet per day will probably soon be realised even for patients with very severe hypertension.

Will the cause of high blood pressure ever be found?

One addage in medical research is 'never say never'. However, it does seem likely that high blood pressure is not a single-factor disease. If a single virus or bacteria causing hypertension is discovered or if it is convincingly shown that the problem is due to poisoning by some insecticide or mineral from the soil, I shall cheerfully eat my hat in public. As I have explained earlier, much the most likely explanation is that there are several factors and that their interplay is largely controlled by patients' inheritance or genetics. Perhaps researchers in the future will be able to define some of these abnormalities more closely. What is also likely to happen is that research into the cause of hypertension will be outflanked by research which goes more directly to the core of the problem, which is why and how does high blood pressure damage blood vessels. If we could stop this damage to blood vessels, then the high blood pressure would be almost irrelevant. Drugs which hold out a promise of regulating some of this attack are already being investigated.

APPENDIX

Medicines used in the treatment of high blood pressure

All the preparations commonly available for the treatment of high blood pressure are included in this table which lists them alphabetically by trade name. The middle column gives the official names of the ingredient drugs and the far column assigns these drugs to one of the various types of drug whose effects and side effects are discussed in Chapter 6. Note that the same drug may be an ingredient of several different tablets and that some tablets contain up to three different drugs.

Proprietary name	Proper name	Drug type
Abicol	Reserpine	Central drug
	Bendrofluazide	Diuretic
Aldactide	Spironolactone	Diuretic
	Hydroflumethiazide	Diuretic
Aldactone	Spironolactone	Diuretic
Aldomet	Methyldopa	Central drug
Apresoline	Hydralazine	Vasodilator
Aprinox	Bendrofluazide	Diuretic
Aquamox	Quinethazone	Diuretic
Baycaron	Mefruside	Diuretic
Berkozide	Bendrofluazide	Diuretic

Proprietary name	Proper name	Drug type
Beta-Cardone	Sotalol	Beta blocker
Betaloc	Metoprolol	Beta blocker
Betim	Timolol	Beta blocker
Blocadren	Timolol	Beta blocker
Brinaldix	Clopamide	Diuretic
Brinaldix K	Clopamide Potassium chloride	Diuretic Potassium supplement
Burinex	Bumetamide	Diuretic
Burinex K	Bumetanide Potassium chloride	Diuretic Potassium supplement
Catapres	Clonidine	Central drug
Centyl K	Bendrofluazide Potassium chloride	Diuretic Potassium supplement
Co-Betaloc	Metoprolol Hydrochlorothiazide	Beta blocker Diuretic
Corgard	Nadolol	Beta blocker
Decaserpyl	Methoserpidine	Central drug
Decaserpyl-Plus	Methoserpidine Benzthiazide	Central drug Diuretic
Declinax	Debrisoquine	Adrenergic drug
Direma	Hydrochlorothiazide	Diuretic
Diumide-K	Frusemide Potassium chloride	Diuretic Potassium supplement
Diurexan	Xipamide	Diuretic
Dopamet	Methyldopa	Central drug
Dryptal	Frusemide	Diuretic
Dyazide	Triamterene Hydrochlorothiazide	Diuretic Diuretic
Dytal	Triamterene	Diuretic
Dytide	Triamterine Benzthiazide	Diuretic Diuretic
Edecrin	Ethacrynic acid	Diuretic
Enduron	Methyclothiazide	Diuretic

Proprietary name	Proper name	Drug type
Enduronyl	Deserpidine Methyclothiazide	Central drug Diuretic
Envacar	Guanoxan	Adrenergic drug
Esbatal	Bethanidine	Adrenergic drug
Esidrex	Hydrochlorothiazide	Diuretic
Esidrex K	Hydrochlorothiazide Potassium chloride	Diuretic Potassium supplement
Eudemine	Diazoxide	Vasodilator
Frusetic	Frusemide	Diuretic
Frusid	Frusemide	Diuretic
Harmonyl	Deserpidine	Central drug
Hydrenox	Hydroflumethiazide	Diuretic
Hydromet	Methyldopa Hydrochlorothiazide	Central drug Diuretic
Hydrosaluric	Hydrochlorothiazide	Diuretic
Hygroton	Chlorthalidone	Diuretic
Hygroton-K	Chlorthalidone Potassium chloride	Diuretic Potassium supplement
Hypertane	Rauwolfia	Central drug
Hypertane Compound	Rauwolfia Amylobarbitone	Central drug Sedative
Hypertane Forte	Rauwolfia Ethiazide Potassium chloride	Central drug Diuretic Potassium supplement
Hypovase	Prazosin	Vasodilator
Inderal	Propranolol	Beta blocker
Inversine	Mecamylamine	Ganglionic blocker
Ismelin	Guanethidine	Adrenergic drug
Ismelin Navidrex K	Guanethidine Cyclopenthiazide Potassium chloride	Adrenergic drug Diuretic Potassium supplement
K-Contin	Potassium chloride	Potassium supplement
Kloref	Potassium salts	Potassium supplement

Proprietary name	Proper name	Drug type
Lasikal	Frusemide Potassium chloride	Diuretic Potassium supplement
Lasix	Frusemide	Diuretic
Lasix K	Frusemide Potassium chloride	Diuretic Potassium supplement
Leo-K	Potassium chloride	Potassium supplement
Loniten	Minoxidil	Vasodilator
Lopressor	Metoprolol	Beta blocker
Metenix	Metolazone	Diuretic
Midamor	Amiloride	Diuretic
Moduretic	Hydrochlorothiazide Amiloride	Diuretic Diuretic
Natrilix	Indapamide	Diuretic
Navidrex	Cyclopenthiazide	Diuretic
Navidrex K	Cyclopenthiazide Potassium chloride	Diuretic Potassium supplement
Nefrolan	Clorexolone	Diuretic
Neonaclex	Bendrofluazide	Diuretic
Neonaclex-K	Bendrofluazide Potassium chloride	Diuretic Potassium supplement
Nephril	Polythiazide	Diuretic
Raudixin	Rauwolfia	Central drug
Rautrax	Rauwolfia Hydroflumethiazide Potassium chloride	Central drug Diuretic Potassium supplement
Rauwiloid	Rauwolfia	Central drug
Rauwiloid + Veriloid	Rauwolfia Veratrum	Central Central drug
Saluric	Chlorothiazide	Diuretic
Saluric K	Chlorothiazide Potassium chloride	Diuretic Potassium supplement
Sando-K	Potassium salts	Potassium supplement
Sectral	Acebutalol	Beta blocker

Proprietary name	Proper name	Drug type
Seominal	Reserpine Theobromine Phenobarbitone	Central drug Alkaloid Sedative
Serpasil	Reserpine	Central drug
Serpasil Esidrex	Reserpine Hydrochlorothiazide	Central drug Diuretic
Slow K	Potassium chloride	Potassium supplement
Slow Trasicor	Oxprenolol	Beta blocker
Sotacor	Sotalol	Beta blocker
Tenoretic	Atenolol Chlorthalidone	Beta blocker Diuretic
Tenormin	Atenolol	Beta blocker
Theogardenal	Phenobarbitone Theobromine	Sedative Alkaloid
Theominal	Phenobarbitone Theobromine	Sedative Alkaloid
Thiaver	Veratrum Epithiazide	Central drug Diuretic
Trandate	Labetalol	Beta blocker
Trasicor	Oxprenolol	Beta blocker
Trasidrex	Oxprenolol Cyclopenthiazide	Beta blocker Diuretic
Vatensol	Guanoclor	Adrenergic drug
Veriloid	Veratrum	Central drug
Veriloid VP	Veratrum Phenobarbitone	Central drug Sedative
Viskaldex	Pindolol Clopamide	Beta blocker Diuretic
Visken	Pindolol	Beta blocker